Quimberlly Oliveira Fernandes
Marcilene Barros

Nurses' view of the Manchester Risk Classification

Quimberlly Oliveira Fernandes
Marcilene Barros

Nurses' view of the Manchester Risk Classification

A survey carried out at a public hospital in Brazil

ScienciaScripts

Imprint
Any brand names and product names mentioned in this book are subject to trademark, brand or patent protection and are trademarks or registered trademarks of their respective holders. The use of brand names, product names, common names, trade names, product descriptions etc. even without a particular marking in this work is in no way to be construed to mean that such names may be regarded as unrestricted in respect of trademark and brand protection legislation and could thus be used by anyone.

Cover image: www.ingimage.com

This book is a translation from the original published under ISBN 978-613-9-72173-3.

Publisher:
Sciencia Scripts
is a trademark of
Dodo Books Indian Ocean Ltd. and OmniScriptum S.R.L publishing group

120 High Road, East Finchley, London, N2 9ED, United Kingdom
Str. Armeneasca 28/1, office 1, Chisinau MD-2012, Republic of Moldova, Europe
Printed at: see last page
ISBN: 978-620-7-94121-6

DEDICATORY:

We dedicate it to God, our parents, our spouses, our siblings and relatives;

To those who have passed on: our tributes and

Miss you.

ACKNOWLEDGEMENTS

To God for giving us the health and strength to overcome difficulties.

To this university, its teaching staff, management and administration, who have provided the window through which I can now glimpse a higher horizon, full of confidence in the merit and ethics present here.

To our supervisor Elizabeth Dreyer, for her support in the short time she had, for her corrections and encouragement.

To our parents, for their love, encouragement and unconditional support.

And to everyone who directly or indirectly played a part in our education, thank you very much.

"For since ancient times there has not been heard, nor perceived with the ear, nor seen with the eye, a God besides you who works for him who hopes in him. "

(Holy Bible - Isaiah 64:4)

SUMMARY

Introduction: Urgent and emergency services are a gateway for users to try to resolve or alleviate their suffering, which is why these sectors are overloaded with high demands. The Manchester Risk Classification was used for the first time in Brazil in 2008. This classification is based on the client's signs and symptoms to classify them according to their severity, leaving behind the old first-come, first-served system. This increased the level of stress in the emergency networks of all hospitals, while also increasing the number of deaths in the queue and the workload for nurses and their teams. The protocol was implemented in the SUS with the aim of decongesting these units in order to offer users differentiated care, and the role of nurses in these units is of great importance for the effectiveness of the protocol. **Aim:** The aim of this study was to analyse nurses' views on the applicability and effectiveness of the Manchester protocol in a hospital in Recife. **Methodology:** This is a quantitative field study, using an interview with direct questions. The study was carried out with 21 nurses working in the emergency department of the Getúlio Vargas Hospital, Recife, in November 2017. **Results and Discussions:** After analysing the data, it could be seen that most of the interviewees were female (95.24%), the highest age range was between 31 and 50 years (66.67%), and 66.67% of the interviewees held specialist qualifications. According to the interviewees, the study shows that the protocol is a working tool that gives nurses autonomy, is a tool for humanising the emergency service, and is effective according to its objectives and mission. However, it is possible to understand that the training carried out by the SUS is still not enough to implement the protocol in the service. **Considerations:** It is therefore considered that the PNH's proposal to implement the Protocol in the public health network is effective, and that systematisation in the emergency sector continues with improvements in care for SUS users.

KEYWORDS: Nursing. Manchester Protocol. Risk classification.

SUMMARY

CHAPTER 1	**7**
CHAPTER 2	**10**
CHAPTER 3	**11**
CHAPTER 4	**17**
CHAPTER 5	**19**
CHAPTER 6	**30**
CHAPTER 7	**31**
CHAPTER 8	**35**
CHAPTER 9	**39**

CHAPTER 1

INTRODUCTION

The demand for urgent and emergency care has grown significantly in recent years, making this sector an important part of healthcare provision (CAVEIÃO et al; 2014).

The growing demand for urgent and emergency services can interfere with the quality of care provided, as it requires more physical and human resources, which are not always available, resulting in queues and waiting times for care (MAFRA et al; 2005).

With the aim of improving care in these units, the Unified Health System (SUS) created a new contemporary health policy in 2003, the National Policy for the Humanisation of Care and Management (PNH) (BRASIL et al; 2010).

The experiment by first world countries to reverse the pattern of their healthcare system in the 1990s coincides with the origin of the first systematised emergency risk classification protocols. These classification models vary widely; there are models that use from two levels to five levels of risk, with the five levels being the most widely accepted today. There are five of the most advanced risk classification models, which have come to have a systemic vision, i.e. they are used by service networks.

The most relevant models are The *Australasian Triage Scale (ATS)* - was the forerunner and uses waiting times according to severity;The *Canadian Triage Acuity Scale (CTAS)* - is more complex than the previous model and is in use in a large part of the Canadian system. The Manchester Model *(Manchester Triage System - MTS)* - works with algorithms and key discriminators, associated with waiting times symbolised by colours. It is used in several European countries. The entry mechanism is a patient's complaint or presenting situation; The American Model *(Emergency Severity Index - ESI)* - works with a single algorithm that focuses more on the need for care resources. It is not used throughout the country; The Andorra *Model (Model Andorrà del Tríalge - MAT)* - It is based on symptoms, discriminants and algorithms but is complex and slow to use (CORDEIRO JÚNIOR et al; 2014).

In this sense, it is believed that the implementation of a more advanced patient assessment system will help to improve the quality of risk classification; organise the flow; guarantee everyone care and access compatible with their needs; and improve and systematise care by assigning clinical priorities (ULHÔA et al; 2010).

The method used by the Ministry of Health for this risk classification and user reception was the Manchester Protocol, which is based on the patient's main complaint and thus classifies them into priority levels, stratifying the risk of each occurrence into five different colour levels for each service: red - emergent; orange - very urgent; yellow - urgent; green - not very urgent; blue - not urgent (ULHÔA et al; 2010),

Within the multi-professional team, nurses take on the role of commanding the flow of patients and their search for care in emergency services, favouring a reduction in morbidity and mortality (ACOSTA, DURO & LIMA et al; 2012).

According to Almeida and Alves (2013), the nurse's duties in the emergency department involve listening to the patient's history, physical examination, providing treatment, counselling patients and coordinating the nursing team. Combining scientific knowledge with leadership skills, agility, quick thinking and the need to remain calm.

Risk classification differs from the traditional concept of triage, since in traditional triage there can be exclusions, while in risk classification all clients will be attended to. The risk classification triage room is a mandatory physical area in emergency care units. Its main purpose is to identify priorities. It is essential in any emergency service (ALBINO et al; 2007).

The implementation of reception with risk classification is synonymous with a change in work organisation, achieving a new guideline for the institution, offering users differentiated care from health professionals. This is expected to reduce queues and improve user care (GOULART et al; 2013).

The implementation of reception with risk classification is synonymous with a change in work organisation, achieving a new guideline for the institution, offering users differentiated care from health professionals. This is expected to reduce queues and improve user care (GOULART et al; 2013).

1.1 BACKGROUND

It consists of the importance of the professional nurse as the gateway to users in urgent and emergency services, following the National Humanisation Policy through the risk classification system adopted, the Manchester Protocol. The stimulus for studying this subject was the interest in nurses' perceptions of the effectiveness and applicability of the Protocol in their service. Taking into account the knowledge and application of this tool as an optimisation of their work, in order to get to know the reality between the theory and the application of the Manchester Protocol, which aims to reduce the waiting time for users, providing fast, quality care, without crowds in this sector that is overloaded with great demands, especially in the SUS. The nurse is the professional at the head of this risk categorisation flowchart, so what is the nurse's view of using the Manchester Risk Classification Protocol as a working tool?

CHAPTER 2

OBJECTIVE

2.1 GENERAL OBJECTIVE

To analyse how nurses work with the Manchester protocol in an emergency hospital.

2.2 SPECIFIC OBJECTIVES

- Identifying nurses' views on the protocol and humanisation in the risk classification process.
- To analyse the applicability and effectiveness of the protocol in the emergency department.
- Characterising the Manchester protocol according to the perception of professional nurses.

CHAPTER 3

THEORETICAL BACKGROUND

3.1 History

Risk classification began in the Napoleonic Wars (1799-1815), when French combatants separated the most seriously wounded. In the Crimean War, in 1854, Florence Nightingale separated patients according to their treatment and the severity of their cases. In the 1950s and 1960s, civilian hospitals in the United States began to work with risk classification, which until then had only been a military activity. And in 1962, nursing was introduced, and it ceased to be just a medical competence, generating conflict between them, but serving as a model for other services (ANZILIERO, 2011).

In 1994, the Manchester Risk Classification Group was set up in the United Kingdom, made up of doctors and nurses working in emergency services, due to the need to establish a consensus among these professionals on how to carry out risk classification. The group's objectives were to standardise triage, including common nomenclatures and definitions, develop a solid triage methodology, plan and implement a training programme and develop an audit guide for triage. Based on studies carried out by the group on existing protocols, the Manchester Triage System was developed (GRUPO BRASILEIRO DE CLASSIFICICAÇÃO DE RISCO, [200-]; MACKWAY-JONES et al, 2010).

Still in the 1990s, some triage models became established internationally, such as the Manchester Triage System (1997), and nationally, such as the Canadian Triage Scale (1999), the Australian Triage Scale (2000) and the American scale - *Emergency Severity Index* (2000), and influenced *emergency* services (ANZILIERO, 2011).

3.2 **Australasian Triage Scale (ATS)**

The Australian Triage Scale is applied in first world countries. They are based on a five-level scale, assigning time and severity, with each level represented by a colour. Triage is carried out by nurses, and clinical descriptors are used to assign the degree of urgency (SANTOS FILHO, 2013).

Category 1 immediate risk to life - immediate care

Category 2 imminent risk to life - 10 minute response time

Category 3 potentially life-threatening care within 30 minutes

Category 4 potentially serious patients - 60-minute service

Category 5 less urgent patients - service within 120 minutes

3.3 **Canadian Emergency Parliamentary Acuity Scale (CTAS)**

Based on the Australian scale, the Canadian Association of Emergency Physicians (CAEP) developed the Canadian Scale. Since its publication in 1999, it has been widely used in Canadian emergency services (ANZILIERO, 2011).

The CAEP always reviews the CTAS, taking into account variables such as workload in emergencies, adapting it to the entire population. The CTAS makes an objective assessment, classifying patients into their priorities and establishing degrees of priority through complaints and modifiers that help in the correct classification of the level of care (ANZILIERO, 2011).

1° order - highest number of complaints (respiratory distress, haemodynamic stability, level of consciousness, fever and severity of pain).

2nd order - limited number of complaints (decrease in glucose, which applies to three complaints: level of consciousness, confusion and hypoglycaemia).

Based on this result, the patient is given a level of care using colours:

Level 1: resuscitation - blue

Level 2 emergency - red

Level 3 urgent - yellow

Level 4: not very urgent - green

Level 5: not urgent - white

3.4 American Triage Scale - Emergency Severity Index (ESI)

Its first version was devised in 1999 and has been used ever since. Care is prioritised through a flowchart assessing the appropriate resources for care. The use of resources is estimated, predicting possible hospitalisation immediately after triage. The ESI works with five levels of severity, from 1 to 5, with "1" being the most serious, requiring immediate intervention. Patients at high risk, disorientated, drowsy, confused, in acute pain and with compromised vital signs are classified as level 2. Patients classified as level 3 to 5 wait safely for a few hours (SANTOS FILHO, 2013).

-Level   1 emergent - immediate assessment;

-Level   2 urgent - 10 minutes until service;

-Level 3 - acute illness, factors do not indicate risk;

-Level   4 - patients with a chronic illness that does not threaten the functions of vital organs;

-Level   5 - stable patients.

3.5Manchester Triage System (MTS) protocol

This protocol classifies patients into five priority levels: level 1 - patients with emergent demands for care and who need immediate medical assessment; level 2 - patients with very urgent demands and who need to be seen within 10 minutes; level 3 - patients with urgent demands who should be seen within 60 minutes; level 4 - patients with less urgent problems who can be seen within 120 minutes; and level 5 - patients who have no urgent demands, and who can wait up to 240 minutes for care, represented by the colours red, orange, yellow, green and blue, respectively (MACKWAY-JONES et al, 2010).

3.6 Classification Flowchart

The Manchester Protocol states that a patient's clinical situation may worsen while they are waiting for medical assessment, which is why the

The priority of care can be altered by a second assessment (GRUPO BRASILEIRO DE CLASSIFICICAÇÃO DE RISCO). Prioritisation of care is based on the patient's complaint and follows 52 flowcharts for the different problems presented. The flowcharts are made up of discriminators, which can be categorised as general and specific. Discriminators are the signs and symptoms that differentiate between the possible priorities, establishing the order of care according to their severity. (SANTOS FILHO, 2013)

General discriminators are those applied to all patients and are independent of their clinical conditions, such as: imminent risk of death, pain, presence of haemorrhage, state of consciousness and temperature. Specific discriminators are applied individually and specifically, related to the characteristics of the clinical condition presented by the patient (COUTINHO et al; 2012). It is important to emphasise that the classification made using the Manchester Protocol is a dynamic process, and it may be necessary to reassess the clinical priority during the patient's waiting time for medical attention, regardless of the severity pre-established by the use of the flowcharts

(COUTINHO et al; 2012).

3.7 Dynamics and Application of the Manchester Protocol

According to Jimenez (2003), risk classification must be carried out by trained and qualified professionals in a suitable environment. It is important that the risk classification time is short in order to maintain its main objective: to guarantee the safety of patients waiting for their first medical attention. According to the same author, the structuring of risk classification takes into account control mechanisms in relation to the areas of the emergency service, as well as the waiting areas. In this way, risk classification becomes a valuable tool for helping to manage care in the emergency service, collaborating with the efficiency of the service and organising the queue fairly, according to the severity of the patient (JIMENEZ, 2003).

3.8 The   Nurse's Role in Risk Classification

Nurses have been appointed to assess and classify the severity of those seeking emergency services, playing an important role in regulating the demand for care and determining the priority of care for these patients (SOUZA et al; 2013). Assigning a degree of risk to a patient is a complex decision-making process and many triage scales have been developed to guide nurses' assessments (BULLARD et al; 2008; ALBINO et al; 2007). Classification protocols allow different assessors to carry out a clinical investigation following the same parameters to establish the severity of patients, which reduces the subjectivity bias of each assessor's view (SOUZA et al; 2013).

The duties of the emergency nurse range from listening to the patient's history, physical examination, carrying out treatment, counselling patients, to coordinating the nursing team, combining scientific knowledge and leadership skills, agility and quick thinking and the need to remain calm (ANDRADE et al; 2000). The generalist characteristics of nurses enable them to carry out nursing consultations, classify and refer patients to the most appropriate clinical area, as well as supervising members of the nursing team, according to COREN, 2010.

CHAPTER 4

METHODOLOGY

4.1 TYPE OF STUDY

The research was carried out on the premises of the emergency department, which has a risk classification room consisting of a table, stretcher, chairs, computer, a Manchester Protocol book; a green, female and male area; a red area; a yellow area; and the corridor, which is also considered a department. The research population consisted of twenty-one nurses from a public hospital in the city of Recife - PE, where the Manchester Protocol was being used as a risk classification system in the emergency department.

The data collection instrument was developed for this research by the researchers themselves with the aim of identifying nurses' knowledge, perception and application of this tool (Manchester Protocol) (Appendix A). Data collection took place in November 2017. The data collection instrument used was a questionnaire with nurses. The answers were tabulated in Excel version 2007. The study followed the guidelines of Resolution 466/2012 of the National Health Council, which regulates the standards applied to research that directly or indirectly involves human beings.

Prior to the fieldwork, the research project was submitted to the Research Ethics Committee - CEP/FUNESO, which issued a favourable opinion on 17/11/2017, according to the copy in Annex B.

4.2 RESEARCH CLASSIFICATION CRITERIA

4.2.1. Inclusion criteria:

Nurses who are part of the Getúlio Vargas Hospital emergency department.

4.2.2. Exclusion criteria:

Nurses who are on holiday or on sick leave; Professionals who do not agree to take part in any stage of the data collection process.

CHAPTER 5

RESULTS AND DISCUSSIONS

The contents of the data analysis were organised into three thematic categories as follows: The profile of nurses working in the HGV emergency department; knowledge of the Manchester risk classification protocol; and the application and effectiveness of the Manchester Protocol in the service;

5.1 The Profile of Nurses Working in the Emergency Department of the Getúlio Vargas Hospital (HGV)

The results presented in Table 1, regarding the characterisation of the profile of the nurses studied, show that 94.12% (n=16) of the professionals interviewed are female; the age group of 31 to 40 years registered the highest frequency 41.18% (n=7), followed by 41 to 50 years adding up to 29.41% of the interviewees (n=5); the predominant marital status was married, with a frequency of 70.59% of the nurses (n=12), followed by single people adding up to 23.53% (n=4).

In 2013, a survey carried out by the Oswaldo Cruz Foundation (FIOCRUZ) and the Federal Nursing Council (COFEN) also highlighted this discrepancy between the female sex, which accounted for 87.3 per cent, and the male sex, with only 11.6 per cent of all nursing professionals in Pernambuco. This research, unlike the present study, showed a slight difference in the frequency of single nurses (42 per cent) and married nurses (41 per cent). With regard to the age of these nurses, it is more frequent between 26 and 40 years old, totalling 56.8%.

With regard to qualifications, it was found that the majority of professionals were specialists (64.71 per cent (n=11)), followed by those with only undergraduate degrees (29.41 per cent (n=5)).

It was noted that most of the group has worked in emergency care for between 1 and 10 years, with 64.71 per cent of those interviewed (n=11), and therefore those with more than 11 consecutive years working in the emergency department, 29.41 per cent (n=5).

These data are also confirmed when analogised with the study by Furtado and Araújo Júnior (2017), which was carried out in a public hospital in Recife, with the aim of finding out about working conditions in the emergency department, based on the perception of nurses working in this sector. The majority of the 23 professionals interviewed were female (91.3%); the predominant marital status (60.9%) was married. It was found that 87% of those interviewed had a specialisation or residency; and 47.8% had been working in the Emergency Department for more than 16 consecutive years.

Table 1 - Socio-professional profile of nurses working in the Getúlio Vargas Hospital emergency department. Recife - 2017.

Variables	Nurses	
	n°	**%**
Sex		
Female	20	95,24
Male	01	4,76
Age group		
21 -30	05	23,81
31 -40	07	33,33
41 -50	07	33,33
51 or more	02	9,52
Marital status		
Single	04	19,05
Married	15	71,43
Divorced	01	4,76
Stable	01	4,76
Titling		
Graduation	05	23,81
Specialisation or Residency	14	66,67
Master's Degree	02	9,52
Working Time in the Emergency Department		
1 to 12 months	02	9,52

| 1 to 10 years | 11 | 52,38 |
| 11 years or older | 08 | 38,10 |

5. 2Knowledge of the Manchester risk classification protocol

When looking at knowledge of the Manchester Risk Classification, it was possible to identify that 76.19 per cent of nurses said they knew the Protocol (n=16), as shown in Figure 1.

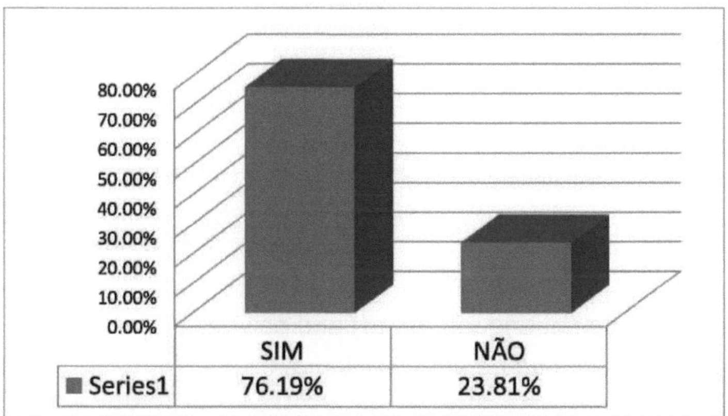

Figure 1. Nurses' knowledge of the Manchester Protocol.

The interviewees were asked if they thought the Manchester Protocol was an important tool in their work, and 100% of the participants confirmed that it was (n=21), as shown in Figure 2.

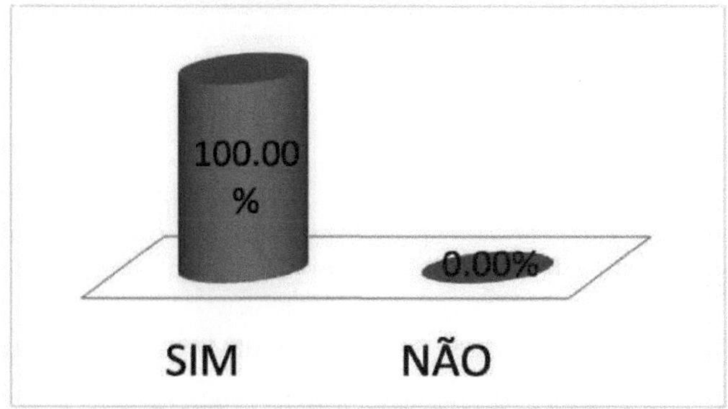

Figura 2.   The protocol as an important working tool

Of the group of interviewees, 52.38 per cent had received specific training on the Manchester protocol, and 47.62 per cent had not, which is equivalent to almost half of the population interviewed, as can be seen in Figure 3.

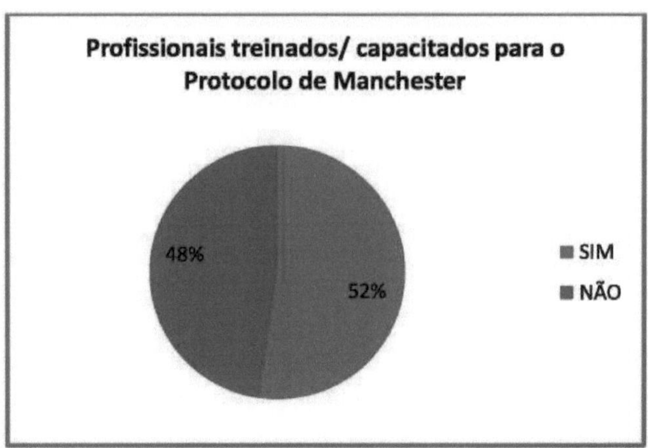

Figure 3: Percentage of professionals trained in the Manchester Protocol. Recife, 2017.

When asked the following question: *"Is the training offered by the SUS enough to implement risk classification in this service?"* 61.90 per cent of the interviewees said it was not enough (n=13) and only 38.10 per cent said it was enough (n=8), which can be seen in Figure 4.

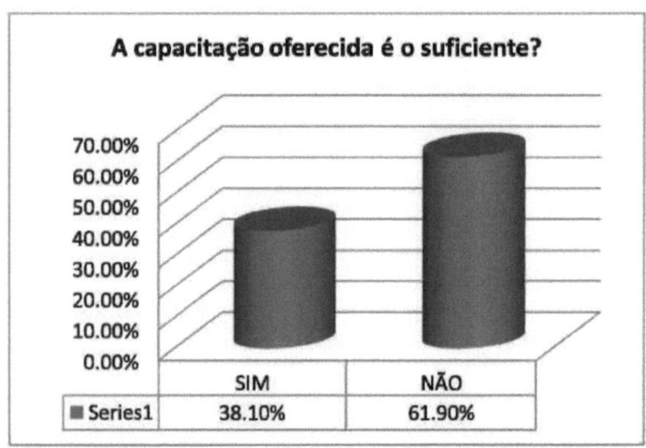

Figura 4.   **Data from the questionnaire: "Is the training offered by SUS enough to implement risk classification?". Recife, 2017.**

Two multiple-choice questions were used in this study's questionnaire to analyse nurses' basic knowledge of the Manchester risk classification protocol. These questions highlighted the relationship between the colour of the severity categorisation and what each colour represents, and the waiting time for care.

The first question listed a patient who had been classified with a red bracelet, and only 38.10% of the interviewees (n=8) correctly answered the alternative: *emergent - immediate, with* the most frequent wrong answer being the alternative: *very urgent - immediate,* representing 42.86% of the group of interviewees (n=9), which is analysed below in Figure 5.

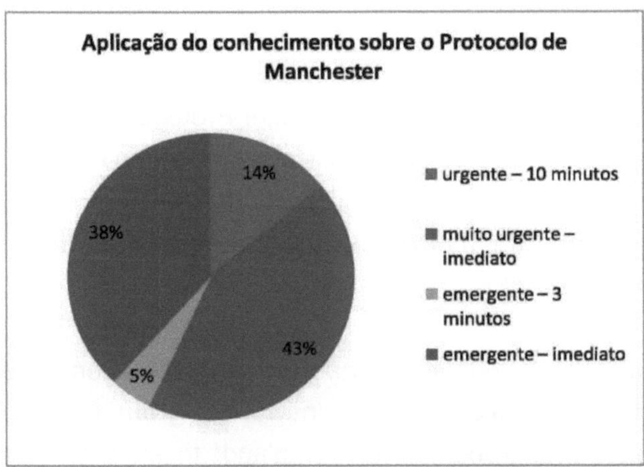

Figure 5: Nurses' knowledge of risk classification.

It can be seen in Figure 6 that the second question listed a patient classified with a yellow bracelet, and the highest frequency was recorded for the correct alternative: *urgent - 60 minutes,* totalling 61.90% of the nurses interviewed (n=13).

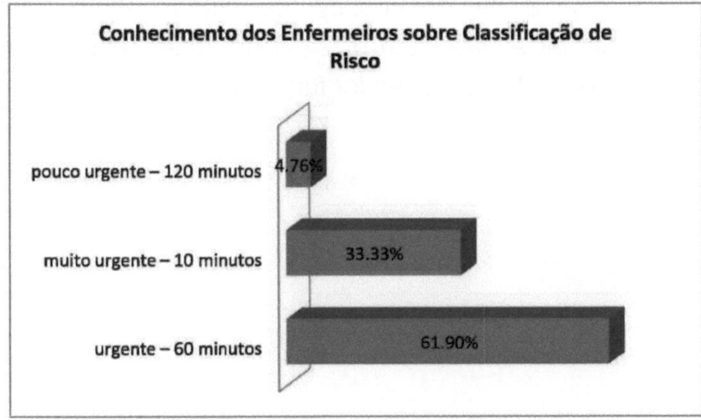

It can be seen that most of the interviewees are familiar with the Manchester protocol, have received training and/or qualification, and all say it is an important tool in their work. However, when asked about the basics of the protocol, it can be seen that most nurses have doubts about the colour - classification - waiting time relationship.

According to Gamara *et al.* (2015), there are currently few national studies on the subject of knowledge about the Manchester Protocol, and even fewer highlighting the role of nurses in the risk classification reception process.

5.3 The application and effectiveness of the Manchester Protocol in the HGV Emergency Department

This study asked some questions about the application and effectiveness of the Manchester Protocol at the institution, given that the protocol is "imported" from a first world country, England, to an emerging country, Brazil, where public health is always pointed out as a scenario of neglect, unhealthy working conditions for professionals, demands are always much higher than what is offered by the SUS, which leads to overcrowding in all sectors of health services. It was observed during the research period that the emergency department was completely overcrowded, so much so that the corridor is considered an emergency area. It was also observed that patients were staying for several days in the emergency department, where it is recommended that they stay for a maximum of 24 hours, after which they should be discharged from hospital or admitted for further treatment.

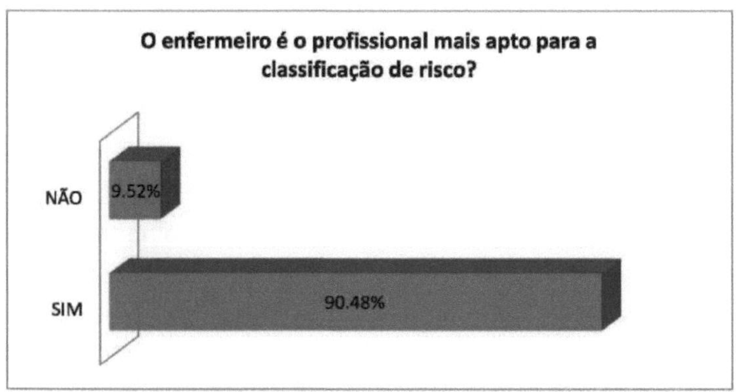

Figure 7.0 nurses consider themselves the most suitable professionals for the Manchester risk classification.

Figure 7 shows that the nurses taking part in the study consider their category to be the professionals best suited to carrying out risk classification, with 90.48% of the interviewees (n=19) agreeing, and only 9.52% disagreeing. This is also evidenced by Shiroma and Pires (2011), in a study aimed at finding out nurses' views on the implementation of Reception with Risk Assessment and Classification in emergency services, which points out that 75% of those interviewed consider that nurses are the most qualified professionals to carry out risk classification, justifying their response based on the association of theoretical and practical knowledge.

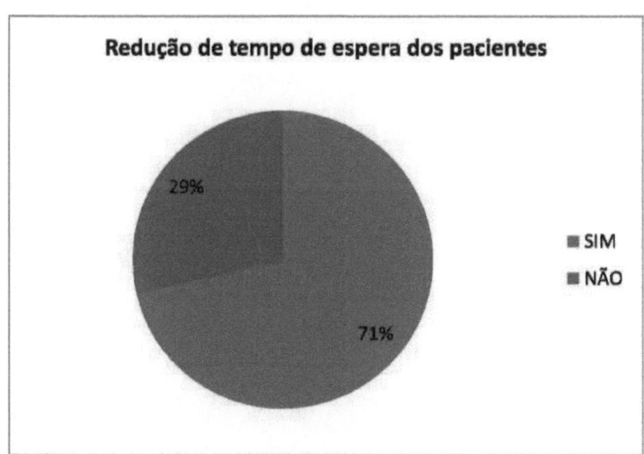

Figure 8. Reduction in waiting time for emergency care at HGV, Recife - 2017.

Figure 8 shows that 71.43% (n=15) of the nurses interviewed believe

25

that implementing the protocol has reduced patient waiting times, while 28.57% (n=6) of those interviewed say that it has not reduced waiting times for service users.

In line with the literature, the study by Oliveira *et al.* (2016), carried out in a hospital in São Paulo, with the aim of identifying whether the time elapsed between risk classification and medical care for less serious patients was in accordance with the institutional protocol, concluded that the average waiting time for medical care did not exceed what is recommended by the emergency service protocol in any of the classification colours.

It was also analysed that 80.95% (n=17) of the interviewees felt that the Manchester risk classification protocol gave nurses greater autonomy, as can be seen in Figure 9 below.

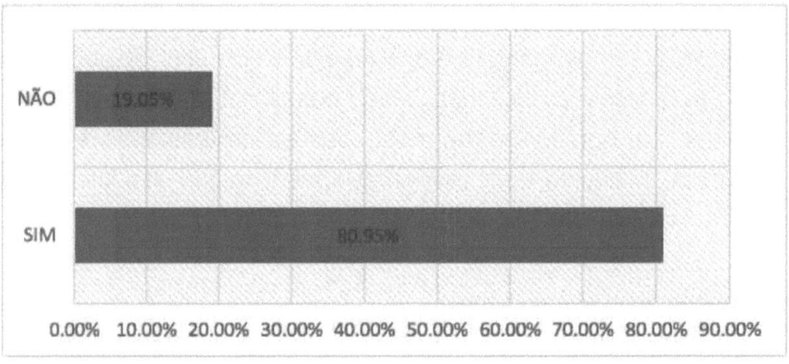

Figure 9. Percentage of interviewees who believe that the Manchester Protocol gives nurses greater autonomy.

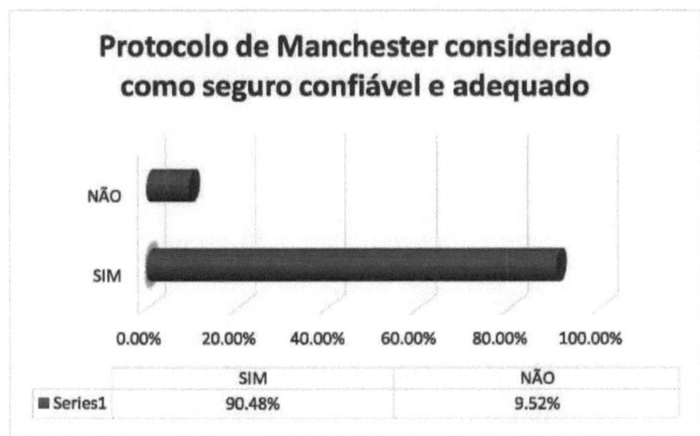

Figure 10. Nurses' perception of the Manchester Protocol.

As analysed above in Figure 10, 90.48% (n=19) of the nurses assessed considered the protocol to be reliable, safe and appropriate. This is in line with the study by Bohn (2013), carried out in a hospital in Porto Alegre, with the aim of analysing the opinion of nurses on the Manchester protocol as a working tool, which points out that the nurses interviewed guarantee that the protocol is safe, as it allows the rapid identification of patients with greater severity at the time of risk classification; it is considered reliable for carrying out structured classification, using the main complaint, followed by the signs and symptoms reported by the user, which follows a flowchart and discriminators, respectively.

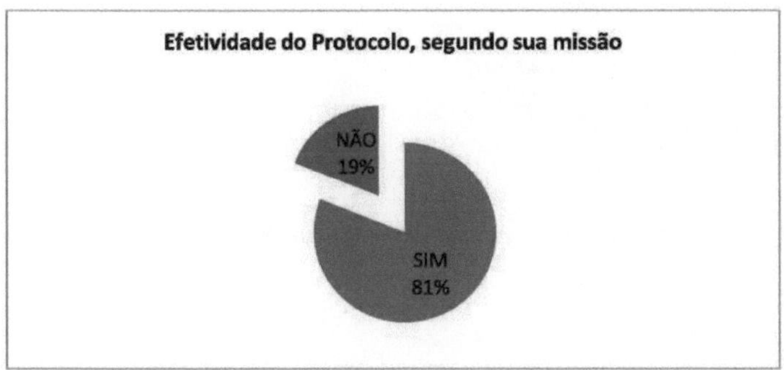

Figure 11. HGV nurses' perception of the Manchester Protocol mission. Recife, 2017.

According to the PNH, the mission of the Manchester Protocol is to welcome the citizen and guarantee better access to urgent/emergency services; to humanise care; and to guarantee fast and effective care, and in relation to this, we were asked whether this mission is fulfilled, according to their perception, and it was analysed that 81% (n=17) of the interviewees positively affirm that the protocol meets its mission, the interviewees who understand that the protocol's mission is not effective, add up to only 19% of the frequency (n=4), this is recorded above, in Figure 11.

In this study, 80.95% (n=17) of the nurses interviewed understood the protocol as a tool for optimising their working time, and only 19.05% (n=4) disregarded it, as shown in Figure 12. According to Bohn in his study (2013), the intention of implementing the protocol is to increase the effectiveness of care, optimise time and resources in services, and increase the satisfaction of users and the healthcare team. Thus, an analogy between the studies shows that the protocol is effective according to its objectives.

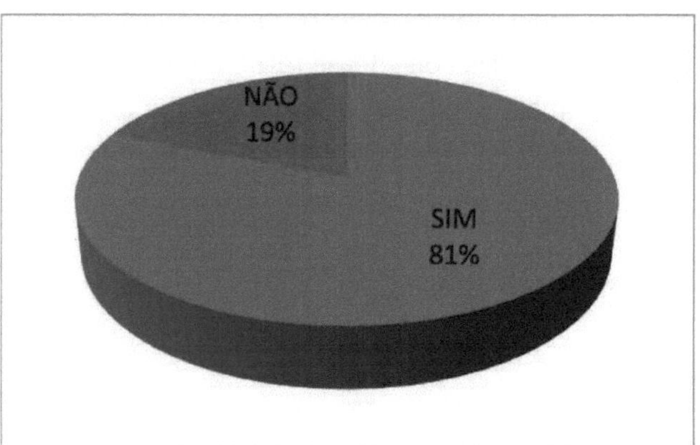

Figure 12. Percentage of nurses who recognise that the Manchester Protocol has optimised their working time

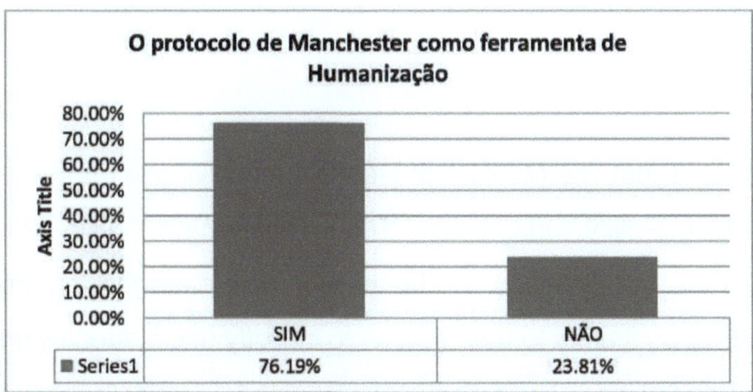

Figure 13. Manchester Risk Classification Protocol, considered a humanisation tool in the SUS urgent and emergency care network.

According to Silva (2014), humanisation in healthcare can be seen as a process, philosophy or way of providing care. Among the various existing conceptualisations, humanisation is expressed in a way of caring for, understanding, approaching, understanding and respecting the patient in moments of vulnerability. According to Figure 13, 76.19% (n=16) of the nurses in this study considered the Manchester Protocol to be a tool that promotes humanisation in urgent and emergency care services.

CHAPTER 6

FINAL CONSIDERATIONS

It is understood that the Ministry of Health's initiative to create the National Humanisation Policy and adopt Risk Classification with the Manchester Protocol as the gateway to the urgent and emergency care network is very positive, as it aims to train nurses to classify users, identifying clinical priority, following the signs and symptoms presented, in order to reduce heavy overloads, and insert the practice of humanisation in this sector.

Its effectiveness can be seen even in the face of the difficulties encountered, such as overcrowding, lack of resources and physical structure, and it is perceived as effective, according to its mission, by the nurses. The use of the Manchester protocol as a working tool for these professionals is quick and straightforward, optimising their working time and giving nurses autonomy. It is safe, reliable and appropriate, as well as being considered an instrument of humanisation, according to the interviewees.

In the view of those interviewed, nurses are the professionals best suited to carrying out risk classification, but they believe that more investment is needed in terms of capacity building/training by the SUS so that implementation can be even more effective.

The Manchester Protocol is therefore considered to be an efficient tool, but there is still a lot of progress to be made, as providing quality care that provides adequate and humanised attention in an environment with so many *deficits* remains a major challenge.

CHAPTER 7

REFERENCES

ACOSTA, AM; DURO, CLM; LIMA, MADS. Nurses' activities in triage/risk classification systems in emergency services: an integrative review, **Rev. Gaúcha Enferm.** vol.33 no.4 Porto Alegre Dec. 2012; available at: http://www.scielo.br/scielo.php?script=sci_arttext&pid=S1983-14472012000400023 [accessed: 23/11/2017].

ALBINO, RM *et al.* Risk classification: an unavoidable necessity in a quality emergency service. **ACM Arq Catarin Med.** 2007;36(4):70-5.

ANDRADE, LM *et al.* **Nurses' perception of the emergency unit.** Ver RENE. 2000; 1 (1):91 -7.

ANZILIERO, F. **Use of the Manchester triage system in risk stratification: literature review. 2011** 47 f. Course Conclusion Work (monograph) - Nursing Course, Federal University of Rio Grande do Sul, Porto Alegre, Rio Grande do Sul. 2011.

BOHN, MLS. **Manchester Risk Classification: the opinion of nurses at the Emergency Department of the Hospital de Clínicas in Porto Alegre.** 2013. 62 f.
Course Conclusion Paper (Monograph) - Nursing Course, Federal University of Rio Grande do Sul, Porto Alegre, Rio Grande do Sul. 2013.

BRAZIL. Ministry of Health. **National Emergency Care Policy** [Internet]. Brasília; 2006 [cited 2013 Dec. 18]. Available from: http://bvsms.saude.gov.br/bvs/publicacoes/politica_nac_urgencias.pdf

BRAZIL. Ministry of Health. **Ordinance no. 2.048, of 5th November 2002. Approves the Technical Regulations for State Urgency and Emergency Systems.** Official Gazette of the Federative Republic of Brazil. 1994 Dec. 15;

BRAZIL. Ministry of Health; Health Care Secretariat. National Policy for the Humanisation of SUS Care and Management. **Reception and risk classification in emergency services.** [Internet]. Brasília; 2009 [cited 2013

Dec. 18].
Available at: http://bvsms.saude.gov.br/bvs/publicacoes/acolhimento_
classification_risk_services_2009. pdf

BULLARD, MJ *et al.* **CTAS National Working Group. Revisions to the
Canadian Emergency Department Triage and Acuity Scale (CTAS): adult
guidelines.**
CJEM. 2008;10(2):136-51.

CAMARA, RF *et al.* The role of nurses in the risk classification process in the
emergency room: a review. **Revista Humano Ser - UNIFACEX,** Natal-RN,
v.1, n.1, p. 99- 114, 2015

CAVEIÃO, C et al. Challenges for nurses in implementing risk classification in
a mixed unit. **Rev Enferm UFSM.** 2014. Jan/Mar;4(1): 189-196.

COREN. Nursing's role in triage with risk classification in emergencies.
COREN-DF Opinion No. 005/2010. Available at:
df.org.brportal/index.php?option=com_contem&view=article&id=684:no-
0052010- atribuiçao-do-profissional-de-enfermagem-na-triagem-com-
classificaçao-de- risconos&catid=38:pereceres&Item=115. Accessed on: 15
March 2013.

CORDEIRO JÚNIOR, W *et al.* **Coordination of urgency and emergency -
SAMU.** Minas Gerais. 233 f. 2008: 48- 49.

CORDEIRO JÚNIOR, W; TORRES, BLB; RAUSCH, MCP. **Manchester Risk
Classification System: Comparing Models.** Brazilian Risk Classification
Group. 2014.

COUTINHO, AAP *et al.* Risk classification in emergency services: a
discussion of the literature on the Manchester Triage System. **Rev Med
Minas Gerais.** 2012; 22(2): 188-198

DIAS, ESS. **Risk classification: Difficulties faced by nurses.**
2014. 27 f. Final course work (monograph) - Nursing Course, Universidade
Federal de Santa Catarina, Florianópolis, Santa Catarina. 2014.

FIOCRUZ; CONFEN. **Research: The profile of nursing in Brazil.** 2015. Available at: http://www.cofen.gov.br/perfilenfermagem/bloco1/tabelas/nordeste/ pe/Enfermeiros.pdf [accessed 23/11/2017].

FURTADO BMASM, ARAÚJO JÚNIOR JLC. Nurses' perceptions of working conditions in a hospital emergency department. **Acta Paul Enferm.** Recife. 2010;23(2): 169-74.

GOULART, CB *et al.* Acolhimento como estratégia para alcançar a integralidade da assistência em hospital de média complexidade. **Semina: Ciências Biológicas e da Saúde,** Londrina, v. 34, n. 1, p. 91-96, jan./jul. 2013.

BRAZILIAN RISK CLASSIFICATION GROUP. **History of Risk Classification.** Belo Horizonte, MG. Available at: http://www.gbacr.com.br

JIMENEZ, JG. **Clasificación de pacientes en los servicios de urgencias y emergencias: Hacia un modelo de triaje estructurado de urgencias y emergencias. Emergencias.** 2003;15:165-174.

MACKWAY-JONES, K; MARSDEN, J; WINDLE, J. **Manchester Risk Classification System. Belo Horizonte: Brazilian Risk Classification Group,** 2010.

OLIVEIRA, GN *et al.* Risk assessment and classification: waiting time for low severity patients. **Rev Enferm UFSM.** Santa Maria. 2016 Jan./Mar.;6(1): 21-28. Available at: https://www.researchgate.net/publication/318611113_Avaliacao_e_ classification _of_risk _waiting_time_of_low_gravity_users [accessed 23/11/2017],

SANTOS FILHO, LAM. **Systematic review of the Manchester Triage System in risk stratification.** 2013. 36 f. Course Conclusion Work (monograph) - Nursing Course. Federal University of Bahia, Salvador, Bahia. 2013.

SHIROMA, LMB; PIRES, DEP. Risk classification in emergencies - a challenge for nurses. **Nursing in Focus.** Santa Catarina. 2011; 2(1):14-17

SILVA, MFN *et al.* Protocol for risk assessment and classification of patients in an emergency unit. **Latin American Journal of Nursing.** Campinas. 2014;22(2):218-25

SILVA, JA. **Humanisation in nursing care for patients in urgent and emergency units.** 2014. 25 f. Course Conclusion Work (monograph) - Nursing Course, Sena Aires Faculty of Science and Education, Valparaíso de Goiás, Goiás. 2014.

SOUZA, CC.; ARAÚJO, FA.; CHIANCA, TCM. Scientific production on the validity and reliability of the Manchester Protocol: an integrative literature review. **Revista da escola de Enfermagem da USP.** Divinópolis. 2015; 49(1): 144-151.

TEIXEIRA, VA.; OSELAME, GB.; NEVES, EB. The Manchester protocol in the single health system and the role of nurses. **Revista da Universidade Vale do Rio Verde.** Três Corações. 2014;12(2):905-920.

ULHÔA M. L. et al. The implementation of new technology: implications for work efficiency in the emergency department of a public emergency hospital. **RGO - Revista Gestão Organizacional,** v. 3, n. 1, Jan- Jun., 2010: 99- 118.

CHAPTER 8

APPENDICES

APPENDIX A - Objective Questionnaire

1. **Age:**
( ) < 20 years
( ) 20 P 30 years
( ) 30P 40 years
( ) 40 P 50 years
( ) 50 or more years old
2. **Level of Education:**
( ) Graduation
( ) Specialist
( ) Master's degree
( ) Doctorate
( ) Post-doctorate
3. **Marital status:**
( ) Single
( ) Married
( ) Divorced
( ) Stable
( ) Widowed
4. **How long have you worked in emergency care?**
( ) 1 to 12 months
( ) 1 to 10 years
( ) 11 years or older
5. **You know the Manchester Protocol**
( ) Yes ( ) No
6. **Have you received specific training on the Manchester protocol?**
( ) Yes ( ) No
7. **Do you think Protocol is an important tool in your work?**
( ) Yes ( ) No

8. **In your opinion, is the Manchester Protocol reliable, safe and appropriate?**
( ) Yes ( ) No

9. **Has the application of this protocol reduced patient waiting times?**
( ) Yes ( ) No

10. **In your opinion, is the nurse the most qualified professional to carry out risk classification?**
( ) Yes ( ) No

11. **Do you see the Manchester protocol as a humanisation tool?**
( ) Yes ( ) No

12. **In your opinion, does the Protocol optimise your working time?**
( ) Yes ( ) No

13. **Do you think the training offered by the SUS is enough to implement risk classification in this service?**
( ) Yes ( )No

14. **Has the Manchester protocol given nurses greater autonomy?**
( ) Yes ( ) No

15. **According to the Manchester protocol, the colours symbolise the estimated time of care and the degree of criticality of the patient. So, what is the classification of a patient signalled with a red bracelet and what is the estimated time for care, respectively?**
( ) urgent - 10 minutes
( ) very urgent - immediate
( ) emerging -3 minutes
( ) emerging - immediate

16. **What is the classification of a patient signalled with a yellow bracelet and what is the estimated time for care, respectively?**
( ) urgent - 60 minutes

( ) very urgent - 10 minutes
( ) emerging - immediate
( ) not very urgent - 120 minutes

17. In his view, the Manchester Protocol is effective, according to its mission: Welcoming citizens and ensuring better access to urgent/emergency services; Humanising care; Ensuring fast and effective service?
( ) Yes ( ) No

8.2 APPENDIX B - Informed Consent Form for those over 18 years of age

Dear Sir, You are being invited to take part in a study, the details of which can be found below. I would like to inform you that you will be interviewed and asked to fill in a questionnaire by the researcher on the premises . This study will be free of charge for the volunteer interviewee, and all financial costs will be the sole responsibility of the researchers. The volunteer and the researcher will receive a copy of this consent form for their records. Research title: NURSES' VIEW OF THE MANCHESTER PROTOCOL IN A RECIFE HOSPITAL. Ethics and Research Committee of the Fundação Superior de Olinda - FUNESO phone (81) 3099-1660. General objective of this research: To analyse the role of nurses in the Manchester protocol in an emergency hospital in Recife. Possible risks of this research: This research offers minimal risk to professionals, and may cause embarrassment when answering the questionnaire, but anonymity is guaranteed. I, ______(full name), the undersigned, declare that I have understood the information contained in this Consent Form, and that all my questions regarding the study and my participation in it have been answered satisfactorily. I freely give my consent to participate as a volunteer in the aforementioned research project. I will answer the questionnaire clearly and truthfully. I reserve the right to discontinue my participation in the study if I deem it appropriate, at any time, without any penalty. All measures will be taken to ensure the privacy and confidentiality of my personal data and the information collected, and it is guaranteed that the results obtained through the research will be used for teaching and research purposes, with the aim of achieving the objectives of the work set out above, including publication in specialised scientific literature and presentation at scientific events.

Recife, //2017   .

____

Participant's signature

Researcher's signature

CHAPTER 9

ANNEXES

ANNEX A - Letter of Consent

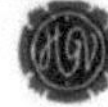 Secretaria de Saúde do Estado de Pernambuco
HOSPITAL
Getúlio Vargas

 OUTUBRO/2017

CARTA DE ANUÊNCIA

Informamos aos interessados que o projeto de Pesquisa intitulado: "A VISÃO DO ENFERMEIRO SOBRE A APLICABILIDADE E EFETIVIDADE DO PROTOCOLO DE MANCHESTER EM UM HOSPITAL DO RECIFE" Será desenvolvido no Hospital Getúlio Vargas – HGV SUS-PE pela pesquisadora, Marcilene Francisca de Barros, Quimberlly de Oliveira Fernandes, Curso de Bacharelado em Enfermagem. sob orientadora Profª Espc. Elizabeth Dreyer.

Informamos ainda que a anuência desta Unidade de Saúde ao Projeto em questão fica condicionada a aprovação do Comitê de Ética em Pesquisa, e que ofereceremos o apoio ao alcance de nossa Instituição.

Recife, 06 de Outubro de 2017.

Dra. Elizabeth Klaus
Coordenadora da COREME/HGV
Gerente do CEAP/HGV
Mat.230419-8

Dr. Gustavo Souza Leão
Diretor do HGV

EKW/kbsb

Av. Gal. San Martin s/n – Cordeiro
Recife – PE - CEP. 50.630-060
Fone: 0XX.81.3184.5600
E-mail: hgvsec@saude.pe.gov.br

ANNEX B - Opinion letter from the Ethics Committee

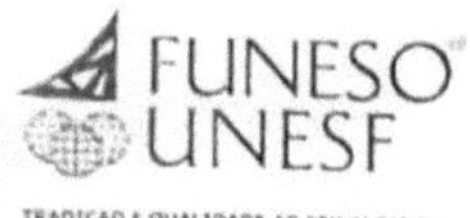

FUNDAÇÃO DE ENSINO SUPERIOR DE OLINDA – FUNESO
UNIÃO DE ESCOLAS SUPERIORES DA FUNESO – UNESF

Comitê de Ética em Pesquisa – CEP/FUNESO
Registro Nº. 1146/2003 – CONEP/CNS/MS

Olinda, 16 de Novembro de 2017

Prezados (as) Pesquisadores (as):

MARCILENE FRANCISCA DE BARROS
QUIMBERLLY DE OLIVEIRA FERNANDES

Nº DO PARECER: 2.382.237

O Comitê de Ética em Pesquisa - CEP/FUNESO, em **Reunião Extraordinária Ordinária no dia 17 de Novembro de 2017**, considerou **APROVADO** o Projeto de CAAE Nº. 79917417.4.0000.5194, intitulado **"A VISÃO DO ENFERMEIRO SOBRE A APLICABILIDADE E EFETIVIDADE DO PROTOCOLO DE MANCHESTER EM UM HOSPITAL DO RECIFE"**. Cujo Objetivo Geral: **Analisar a atuação dos enfermeiros sobre o protocolo de Manchester em um hospital de Emergência**. E tem como Pesquisadora Principal **ELISABETH SANTIAGO DREYER**.

RESUMO DO PARECER DO CEP

O estudo não apresenta riscos e agravos bioéticos e está em consonância com a Resolução 466/12 do Conselho Nacional da Saúde.

Atenciosamente,

Profa. Eva Maria da Silva
Coordenadora - CEP/FUNESO/UNESF
Mat. 20141

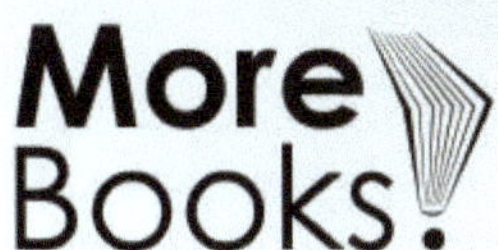

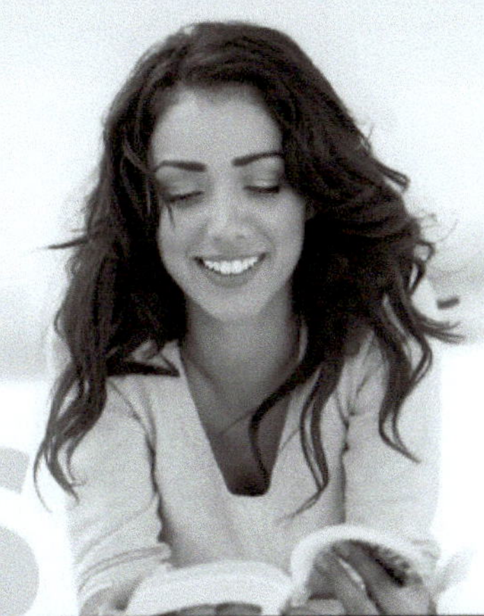

yes

I want morebooks!

Buy your books fast and straightforward online - at one of world's fastest growing online book stores! Environmentally sound due to Print-on-Demand technologies.

Buy your books online at
www.morebooks.shop

Kaufen Sie Ihre Bücher schnell und unkompliziert online – auf einer der am schnellsten wachsenden Buchhandelsplattformen weltweit! Dank Print-On-Demand umwelt- und ressourcenschonend produziert.

Bücher schneller online kaufen
www.morebooks.shop

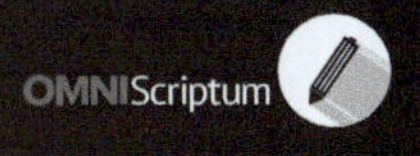

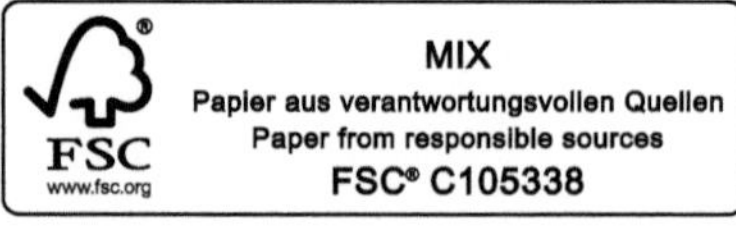